CW01499154

AGAI
THE ODDS

A MOTHER'S LEGACY OF STRENGTH

DEEPAK SHUKLA

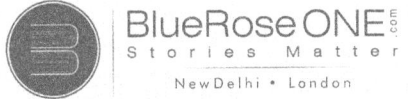

BlueRose ONE
Stories Matter
NewDelhi • London

BLUEROSE PUBLISHERS
India | U.K.

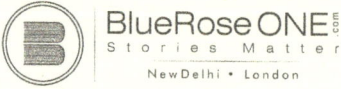

For permissions requests or inquiries regarding this publication, please contact:

BLUEROSE PUBLISHERS
www.BlueRoseONE.com
info@bluerosepublishers.com
+91 8882 898 898
+4407342408967

ISBN: 978-93-6783-443-5

Cover design: Shivam
Typesetting: Namrata Saini

First Edition: December 2024

Contents

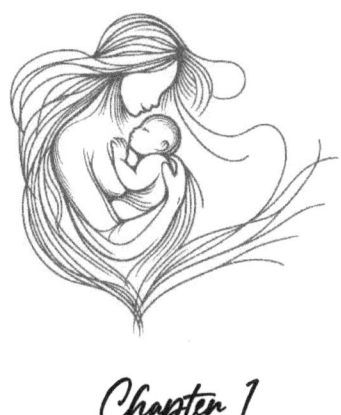

Chapter 1

Resilience in Adversity

What our parents do for us is hard to express in words. The little things we learn, observe, and experience just by being with them shape us into the people we become. Like most of us, how I lead my life today has been hugely influenced by my mother, Daya. It's truly incredible to witness how a mother goes the extra mile, often sacrificing her own pleasures and needs to ensure her children achieve everything they deserve and more. My mother Daya was no different. However, what sets her apart is how she brought us through the adversities life threw at us and led us to the stairs of success.

It's impossible to describe everything a mother does for her children, but as we navigate the complexities of today's world, simple stories like these serve as inspiration for generations. This story is an attempt by a son to share how his mother laid the foundation for his future and how her lessons continue to inspire and influence the way he leads his life today.

There lived a woman named Daya Shukla in the lively town of Meerut, in the northern state of Uttar Pradesh in India. Her life was no different from many other women of her generation in her community: a series of repetitive cycles of family and tradition. She was a complete family woman; married to Jai Prakash, a mother of three children: Preeti, Priya, Deepak – and being a good homemaker. For years, she had played her part as the dutiful wife, content in her bubble, though she was fully aware of the struggles of running a home on the husband's income. However, life, as it would turn out, had a different fate in store for her.

It was February 2001, a month that started with joy and dancing in her mother's village in Gonda, Uttar Pradesh. For two wedding ceremonies in a family, relations arrived in droves singing and dancing while adorning the ceremonies with colourful attires. My mother was there too, helping in her own way to prepare everything as per the plan and to the best of her ability. My father, Jai had remained behind in Meerut expecting to be with her sometime later. But fate intervened.

One morning, while the preparation for the celebration was in progress, a phone call came, interrupting all the fun. My father had met with a severe accident while on his way back from his workplace. The man's voice was serious and every time he said something, it was as though an age passed. My mother's heart dropped, and a wave of cold fear washed over her. At that moment, she felt like a switch had been thrown, and her life was going to turn in a very different direction. Without any delay or second thought, she abandoned the celebrations and ran back to Meerut.

The journey back was heartbreaking. On average, Gonda is only a few hours away from Meerut, but the time seemed to be endless. Every minute that was gone was spent with anxiety and unspoken hope. When she got to the hospital, she was met with a shocking sight: my father, limp and lifeless, connected to numerous monitoring equipment. Despite the efforts made by the doctors, the injuries were quite grievous. She waited near my father for ten terrible days, expecting the situation to change and praying for a miracle to happen, which was, however, never a possibility. He died, and this left my mother a widow at the age of 38 years.

The days that followed the death of my father were chaotic and full of sorrow and confusion. My mother found herself thrust into a role she had never prepared for the breadwinner and the only hope for her family. People came to the house, cried with the family, and consoled them, but they also inquired about things that my mother could not respond to. "Are you going to get married again?" some wanted to know. "How will you take care of your children?" people asked. She had no answers; all that was within her was emptiness, the vacuum of loss and the looming terror of an unknown future.

It appeared that her whole universe was being turned upside-down. My dad supported the family and looked after all the work, including managing money and the children's studies. He was the provider, the one who made the decisions, the one we looked up to and depended on. Without him, she seemed to be a boat that floats but with no direction or a map to guide it through the stormy waters. She had no experience working outside the home. How was she supposed to go on?

However, with each passing day, she found herself developing a new kind of determination within her. She began to find out that the world had changed, but whatever had happened, she had the power to decide how she would face it. "Will crying bring him back?" she questioned herself. "I have to be strong—for my children." She understood that we were looking at her, waiting for her to teach us how to deal with the fact that our father was no longer alive. If she were to break down, then what would become of us?

The first thing that she did was to make sure that we got on with life as usual. She thought that it was important that we continue with our daily activities so that we could come to terms with the fact that our father was no more. "We will not make any significant changes," she stated. "We will continue as though nothing had happened." She placed us in the same schools, ensured we went to class, and helped us to chase our dreams. It was her attempt to keep the storm that had entered their lives from getting any worse.

However, despite all those outward appearances, she was struggling with her loss, too. She missed my dad, hearing his voice on the phone and the way he tried to cheer her up and make things bearable. When we were fast asleep at night, she would allow herself to cry by letting her tears roll down her cheeks. But in the morning, she would wake up and wash her tears, then face us. "We must learn to live with his memory," she would tell us. "Although his presence is seemingly gone through his physical form, he resides with us spiritually."

Her strength served not only as a strength for us but also for everyone who knew her. People who knew her could not believe how happy she was all the time despite the problems she had to go through. Although she was not one to speak much, her actions were louder than words. In spite of this, she did not allow her situation to overcome her. Instead, she decided to become greater than them, to fight for each day regardless of the situation she was in.

One day, a relative visiting them from another city inquired whether she or we were ever feeling depressed. These words touched a sensitive cord in the heart of my mother. She began to appreciate the fact that she could not just rely on sustaining the immediate needs of the family, but she also had to ensure that we were well mentally and emotionally. "We must rise above sorrow," she said to us. "As individuals we need to support each other and move on."

She started believing in herself and developed a single-handed mission to stay strong. "Don't live a life of sympathy," she would often advise me. "People will give you their condolences, and well, condolences are going to drain you dry. They are not going to help you go very far," They are going to use your feelings; meanwhile, you better use them as your power! She also wanted us to know that life is not always going to be fair, but that was not a reason to give up.

As the months went by, we started emulating her and became strong like our mother. We studied for classes, took care of the household chores and stood by one another when one of us was struggling. Whenever we lacked morale or felt exhausted, she would recall our father's desire to see us achieve success. "He wanted you to be strong," she would say. "He wanted you to succeed," she stated, "Make him proud."

Even when she had so much on her plate, she always knew how to crack a joke. She understood that laughter was an excellent remedy for sorrow. She would be joking around, telling stories, and doing anything to make us happy, even in the midst of difficult times. We were often surrounded by one famous quote that she used: "Laughter is the best medicine." "It helps us distract from our problems, although maybe for only an hour or two."

It was truly incredible how she could always find a positive note in even the most unpleasant of situations. She always looked for the bright side of life; she could laugh even when she felt like there was no hope. It was this optimism, this assurance that things would improve and that life would return to normality that kept her going. And gradually, we also started accepting what she claimed to be true.

Among the most significant issues she struggled with was the ability to take care of the family's financial situation. My dad was the only earning member of the family, and with him gone, money was an issue. The family was living on a small pension, and the little we were able to save over the years. However, she was not ready to let things go that easily and was prepared to find ways of making it work. She, therefore, eliminated unnecessary spending, started saving and knew how to work hard to make her rupee count. "We may not be rich," she would say, "but we are not poor, and we don't need more than we already have."

This was not always the case, and there were some days when the figures did not appear promising—no cash for the rent or to take to the grocery store. But she never allowed us to see how worried she was. She would find a way, she always did. "God will provide" she would smile confidently, with kind of faith that makes a person real. And in some way or another, things always turned out fine.

After several years, she became a symbol of hope not only to her family but also to everybody who knew who she was. Her story went viral across the community to empower those who had challenges to take on by struggling to overcome them. She was the epitome of power, proof that no matter how bleak the future may seem, there is always a way to overcome it.

In her story, one learns that power does not lie in being protected from difficulties but in enduring them. Her ability to stay strong despite unbelievable adversity made us—and everyone who knew her—understand that no matter what life throws at us, we can come out on the other side even stronger if we do not let go.

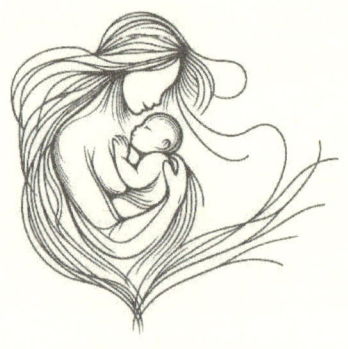

Chapter 2

Embracing Change with Grace

Life is unpredictable. It takes us to places we never wished or wanted to be and transforms us into persons we never envisaged. My mother, Daya, survived such uncertain moments, and her resilience speaks more about her than anything else. She accepted changes with a passion and with full willingness to do whatever is required of her, be it overwhelming. Resilience as she illustrated it, is not merely simply the ability to continue to exist, but to flourish in new challenging and unpredictable environments.

When my father died, the world that my mother had known for close to twenty years was taken away instantly. She had been a homemaker, which she did with pride, realising that my father was there to earn and make decisions on matters such as finances. In many ways, they provided backup for each other – he was the breadwinner, and she was the housewife. But after his death, everything changed, and she woke up one day without her partner, without somebody to count on in many aspects of her life.

For my mother, this entailed having to undertake tasks that she used to think she would never have to do. She had no other option than to take up positions that were new and challenging to her. There were many things to sort out: bills, our education, and, most importantly, the future, and all of that without my father. It was like being thrust into the deep end, and therein one has to fend for themselves in the best way possible. She said that one of the most challenging changes was the fact that now she was the only one to make all the solitary choices that would impact the family.

However, as usual, my mother did not allow herself to back down from the situation. She was not afraid to do what she had to do. However, she did not lose heart and instead demonstrated a level of dynamism that I had not seen in her before. In those early days after the death of my father, I found that my mother had been put through trial after trial over and over again. Among the earliest difficulties she had to face was the need to control the family's finances. My father used to look after the finances, while my mother never worked and had no insight into the finances of the household, savings and debts.

The little pension given to us after the demise of my father did not meet our daily needs, much less our education needs. My mother was forced into managing money, getting the maximum value for every rupee, and making a number of tough calls related to finances. That is why she turned out to be a master at knowing what must be saved for and what has to be eliminated without making us think that we are living a poor life. Sometimes, she did not have many things for herself, but she ensured that we didn't feel the pinch of hardship as far as finances were concerned. Her ability to adapt to this new situation was profound not only in terms of learning how to exist in it but how to thrive in it.

It was not only the financial aspect that brought her to practicality and forced her to change her ways. There were psychosocial changes that accompanied single motherhood in a society where widowed women were frowned upon, especially after the death of their husbands. In our community, people gossiped. They came up with mind-probing questions about whether she would get married again or how she could ensure she was feeding three children. When such questions were being raised, her close friend Subhadra stepped up and gave her the confidence she needed. Subhadra was not only her friend but also, due to the age difference, a coach and a mentor. She had been a close family friend for more than 25 years, and as Daya was recovering from the loss, lacking confidence and in a state of confusion, Subhadra introduced her to the purpose of her life. She ensured that Daya understood that if she had clarity on the purpose of her life, she would be able to deal with such questions, rumours, or whatever better. During the course of discussions over a few weeks, she kept reminding my mother that her focus now really was her children and their future. My mother answered these questions calmly, but she also made it very obvious that her concern was for us, the children, and the future.

Her greatest worry was for her two daughters, Preeti and Priya, who were still in their teens. Raising daughters in our society is not an easy task as it comes with its own unique challenges and pressures. Many people used to tell my mother how she would marry them without my father's support. "Who will marry them now?" they would ask as if the girls would have no future, no hope for acceptable husbands since their father was not around to find them proper matches. My mother, however, never allowed these social norms to guide her choices in her life. She realised that her daughters required education, confidence, and freedom far more than they required early marriages. This was a rather ingenious mindset, particularly at that time. So, without getting influenced by any of these norms, she ensured that both Preeti and Priya continued their schooling in the same school they had been studying at. Children start to accept responsibility as they adapt to situations where opportunities and support are limited. We should also give credit to some goodness that exists in the society. Her decision to continue as-is got support from their school as well, who offered a 50% discount on their annual fees.

My mother's adaptability extended to the pragmatic aspects of our lives. When our financial situation became dire, we faced the difficult decision of downsizing. We adopted a more minimalist lifestyle in our family home, making sacrifices to manage our expenses. However, she understood the necessity of the changes. Despite the challenges, my mother approached this transition with remarkable resilience. Rather than dwelling on what we had lost, she focused on the opportunities ahead. Her ability to see the positive in difficult circumstances was truly inspiring.

As my sisters and I began to grow old, my mother's flexibility was challenged yet again. We were not children anymore who required her attention all the time, and she had to become accustomed to being the mother of young adults with our goals and plans. It was a balancing act. On the one hand, she wanted to take care of us, to go on commanding us as she used to when we were children. On the other hand, she understood that we wanted freedom, we had to decide on something on our own, and we always learned from our errors.

An instance of this was when I showed a desire to attend college. Having done my engineering, I blurted one day that I wished to go for an MBA. At first, I noticed the uncertainty, and I could see that she was struggling with something in her mind. She realised that obtaining an MBA would take time away from when I would be able to stand on my own financially, let alone the high cost of the program. But instead of saying no, my mother had a tendency to change for the worse once again in the situation. She knew the hidden value of an MBA degree, and regardless of her busy schedule, she assisted me in getting the loans I required for the course when I was rejected at first.

This was not only her determination to seek a way of paying for my education; but rather her visions beyond the hurdles. She knew that change was not just for the present, change is about preparing for something more suitable. And that's exactly what she did for us.

I can recall that one of the most beautiful aspects of my mother's transformation was her willingness to learn. Despite the fact that she only went up to the eighth grade in school, she never allowed that to be a hindrance to her. Seeing that she had barely managed to arrange our lives after my father's death, she thought about the fact that she had to gain more knowledge. She also embraced learning about bureaucratic procedures and financial systems of banks and asking friends and families for knowledge in all the areas she had no knowledge of. She didn't shy away from seeking assistance and guidance from her mentors and friends. This proves that flexibility means being teachable and open to development.

She was also flexible in her emotions and that made her realise that no one is infallible. Although my mother has been depicted as a very strong and pragmatic woman from childhood, she did not lose her spirit and knew that it was necessary to remain an emotional woman. She had to shift from one position to another by not only coming to terms with the death of her husband but also being the one to tend to the children's emotional issues. She understood and accepted the fact that each one of us has his or her own way of mourning that is based on his or her timeline. While she was present when one of us needed her, she never overemphasised our emotions, yet she allowed us to deal with them on our own.

While we were all going through this and settling into our lives, she maintained a whole feeling of positivity about my father. She would repeatedly say that he was not here physically but that he was there for us. In the short span of time he had been with us, the amount of love and care he had given was enough for us to live our lives with. Her continuous repetition of all the positives about my father and embedding the thought that with limited resources, we were still able to maintain a similar life as he left us was possible only due to his blessing.

What was remarkable about my mother's flexibility was that she accomplished these tasks seamlessly. She never complained, and she hardly showed signs of frustration. She just kept on going, and no matter what, she continued to soldier on and face the tides of change. For her, even when surrounded by unknowns, she was able to pull through. She respected the uncertainty of life and encouraged everyone to do the same.

She never complained and would say, 'If not this, we'll have some other challenges in life.' Life's never a bed of roses, and yes, in the absence of such an important member of our family, we will have to show strength to come out victorious at the end of this. While she was adapting to the changes in her life, she would keep the three of us motivated by saying that this would make us stronger and give us the resilience to face the hardships life throws at us.

A valuable lesson learned is that sometimes, we need to let bad times pass. As time, days, seasons, and years change, so do situations. Keeping focused on our purpose helps us navigate through them better.

Finally, I realised that my mother provided each one of us, her children, with this beautiful attribute of flexibility and resilience. She proved to us that no matter how things are in life, they are capable of switching, of growing, and of surviving. She showed us that flexibility in life is not just a matter of coping with adversity—it is leveraging adversity to become better. For that, I will forever be grateful.

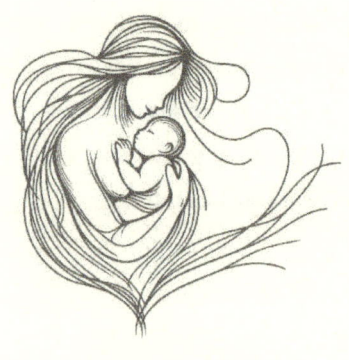

Chapter 3

Strength in Motherhood

Most parents agree with the statement that there are no stronger forces in the universe than a mother's love. It is a love that is without demand, one that endures without complaint, one that is rarely said but felt in every fibre of her being and defines the lives of her children in ways they may not understand until they are adults. My mother, Daya, was an embodiment of this love every day of her life. Her responsibility as a mother was to keep our family together after the shocking death of my father. From her love, strength and determination, my sisters and I were able to move on no matter how hard the journey appeared.

The day my father died, all the burden of life fell on my mother. She was left with three children—two young daughters and a son—to raise on her own. She had never worked, she had never earned a steady income for her, and she was now being presented with a future that was both bleak and daunting. But it is in such a moment, when the woman is grieving, those inherent mom qualities shine through. She didn't permit herself to be downcast for too long as the feelings overwhelmed her. She, therefore, decided to take up the role of both mother and father to us so that we would never miss the father's absence as much as we were receiving what we wanted.

Some of the first lessons my mother put into practice as a widow include keeping our lives as natural as possible after my father's death. Growing up as kids, we were lost, bewildered and devastated. We did not understand how to handle it when our father died. But my mother knew that the worst thing for us to do was to change our habits and do everything possible to maintain our schedules. She made sure that we kept on attending the same schools, engaging in the same activities, and having the same dreams as we had prior to the demise of our father.

"Your education, your future, you cannot afford to be affected," she emphatically refused to let us suffer the sting of the tragedy that had just befallen our family. The decision to stay with the current structure and resist change can be said to have been one of the most strategic choices she made; she possibly appreciated the importance of stability in children's lives, particularly when the world is changing.

But what we failed to grasp at that point was how challenging it was for her to maintain that level of consistency. The truth was, however, that my mother was under enormous stress as a single parent of three young children. We did not witness her tossing and turning as she contemplated how she would be able to feed her family. We were never aware of these struggles she underwent. She would deny herself minor necessities so that we do not feel she is suffering. She endured all of it and never let us know what she was going through or the state she was in.

What was even more inspiring was the fact that my mother was not only strong physically but also emotionally, as she was able to help us even when she was going through so much pain. It was not only physical needs that she met for us; she also took care of us and made us feel wanted and appreciated. I recall how she would sit down with my sisters and me, listening to our complaints and grievances and promising to solve all our issues. She especially had an amazing skill in making me feel protected through a heavy shroud of uncertainty outside.

It seems that in Daya's story, her strength in motherhood was demonstrated through those minor acts of care and support. She had the natural ability to understand when one must be embraced or when one needed to hear some nice words or be listened to. In particular, when my sisters and I had academic problems or could not handle the challenges of growing up, she was always there with kind words of motivation. "You are much tougher than you believe you are," she used to say to us. "It will be okay; it always is. This is just the next challenge for you to face and overcome. "

I see now that she invested so much of herself to nourish our spirits, to create strength within us. She never made any of us think that we were in a worse position because our dad was no longer with us. In fact, she went the extra mile to make sure that we never had the impression that we were missing anything. She would always like to remind us, "Your father is no longer physically present, though his spirit will always remain with us, and I am here. I will be both your mother and your father."

It was not only her encouragement that helped us find strength; it was what she did. I also learned how to be strong and persevere through the difficult situations she was facing in her life. In difficult times, she did not grumble and did not quit. Instead, she was able to endure and look for ways of surmounting all the odds that crossed her way. Of all her abilities, it was very evident that she was a great negotiator when it came to making arrangements for my MBA loan. I had applied for the loan, but it was declined initially; I got home feeling like I could not get a loan anywhere. But my mother has not given up yet. The next day she went to the bank, had a word with the manager of the bank and brought him round to agree to offer her the loan. It was a moment that defined the strength and determination she must have within her; no power in this world was going to prevent her from making sure that her children got whatever they wanted in this world.

This incident was not just about getting the loan; it was about the lesson she taught me: From the biblical sense, the love and affection that a mother has for her children is incomparable and can even make mountains shift. She wasn't just struggling for a loan; she was struggling for my life. And that's what she did every day—she fought for us, no matter how hard things grew to be.

It is crucial to note one of the most constant aspects of my mother – she was a humorous lady. Though she faced many challenges in life, she never failed to turn things around and make us laugh. I believe that, in fact, humour was the only way she could deal with life, and she was able to take everything that came her way, no matter how difficult it was. She used to say that the best antidote to sadness was laughter, so our home was always warm and happy no matter what was going on outside.

The age my mother knew us to be in with my brother and me was when she realised the dynamics of friendship and people around us would largely be the shaper in much of how we thought and developed in life. She befriended most of our friends, a role she played with humour and perception, too. Her sense of humour helped her find smart, indirect ways of learning what was happening in our lives. She would relax and then simply chat with our friends, laugh at times, and, with a subtle twist on a light note, ask about our conversations, thoughts, and college life. That was not snooping—it was her quirky way of observing us, checking if we were headed in the right direction and staying clear of things that had the potential to damage our physical or mental well-being.

Of all the friends I have, it was Mayur who became, for all practical purposes, my mother's "spy" in our circle of friends. He spent a lot of time in our house, talking to my mother, laughing for hours, and innocently divulging all information connected with our group. In his elation and frank nature, Mayur often let loose things that he probably shouldn't have— things that'd get me and some of our friends into rather embarrassing situations. But that was my mother's way—with never an intrusive word, she came to know the other side of us, to learn what company we kept, what influences we faced when she wasn't around.

But most wonderful of all was how much friends adored her. The best friends whom I had regarded, along with my sisters, as close relatives considered her their friend, too. She would bounce ideas off them, test her thoughts on them, and seek to gain a deeper understanding of how the next generation thought— what their aspirations were, what motivated them. She was always curious and always learning, even through these interactions with people far younger than herself. My friends were inspired by what they considered to be conversations with my mother. They found the depth of passion she carried for her children and the time she devoted to every aspect of our lives. But the thing they understood from my mother was her strength—how, amidst the life of loss and the lashes she had to endure as a single parent, she continued to sport a smile, laugh, and really care for us.

Her greatest gift was the ability to connect with people, especially young people, and not only superficially but actively show interest in their lives, dreams, and challenges. And in return, they left our home with a deeper appreciation for the kind of person she was-someone who could look and stay optimistic and even full of humour amidst what her shoulder carried on her. And to them, she wasn't my mother but a fountain of wisdom and strength. Someone who could make them laugh even when life seemed a little tough.

For her, humour was not just a way to cope with life but the mode by which she built relationships and lifted the spirits of people around her. It is in that humour that she navigated the complexities of life, whether when raising children as a single mother or facing her illness with dignity. That humour never wore off, even on the final days. It was a constant light that continued to shine bright as her body grew weaker.

Her laughter was not just a way of shielding herself from the pain; with her, there was always hope that despite everything, life could still be beautiful sometimes. She would call us and sit us round the dining table and narrate stories from her childhood, and we would all laugh till we could hardly breathe. "Laughter keeps us going," she would say. "If one can find a reason to smile, he will find the strength to confront anything, " and this statement proved to be true. We are grateful for the simple things: her ability to find joy even in this difficult circumstance.

Yet, the most evident way my mother displayed strength was in the way she nurtured my sisters. Daughters in today's society face certain burdens and difficulties, especially if they are fatherless. It was evident that people would approach my mother, often asking her how she was going to marry them off — as if that was the only way their lives were going to turn out. But Daya had a dream for her daughters in her eyes. She never wanted them to be spineless people who needed someone to be with them all the time – she wanted them to be strong women who could take care of themselves.

She would say this to my sisters, "You don't need someone to make you complete, you are complete on your own, you can study, work, achieve your dreams and everything will follow." My sisters Preeti and Priya were brought up with this kind of empowerment and they always knew it was alright that they did not fit the cultural norm. And it was all due to our mother's presence and actions.

Daya was determined to make a point that her daughters should never feel as if they were inferior to any other male or female. My mother always ensured that the three of us enjoyed equal treatment in the family. There were days when I had to study for my graduation, while my sister Preeti would earn money at home giving maths tuition to local kids. She would send me the money for my monthly expenses, never making me feel that I should be ashamed of or embarrassed about it. My mother encouraged her daughters by constantly reminding them of the fact that it wasn't only the responsibility of men in the house to take the financial burden; women had to do the same in an equal ratio. She believed in the strength of women to be able to contribute, lead, and help each other when needed.

My other sister, Priya, who was six years younger than me, would still keep an eye on me to ensure that I had all that was required to study well. The roles we played within the family were never determined by gender or age but by the values that my mom instilled in us- that we were all responsible for each other's welfare, success, and happiness. Three women-my mother and sisters-were my pillars. The three stood by me with the confidence that no time would leave me alone or unsupported because behind them was my mother's strength-the strength she derived from her firm belief in equality and mutual respect, very much something she practiced and bequeathed upon us all.

She insisted on purpose on their academic performance, helped them Search for jobs or any job they wished, and would not allow them to say they were inferior because they were women. She understood that the people around us would desire to place some barriers on what we could do, and she made sure that they never got to affect us in our home. Her love was strong, fired up, defence and invincible, something that empowered them; because of that, my sisters have turned into successful and capable women who are ready to fight for their dreams.

Looking back at my childhood and up to adulthood, I can see and feel my mother's strength not only in making us successful in life but also in moulding us to be good-hearted and independent. Looking back, sometimes I wonder—was it just destiny or the strength of my mother's foresight and decisions that I am sitting here in London, advising global businesses on their future growth strategies? There are moments when I reflect on how differently things could have turned out. I could've been working as a government clerk somewhere in an office in Meerut, doing something I never wanted to do, feeling trapped in a life that didn't align with my ambitions. However my mother's unwavering belief in my potential and her constant encouragement to pursue what I truly wanted ensured that I never settled for less than what I was capable of achieving. It's her strength, her vision, and her ability to make tough decisions that have led me to where I am today.

This is why she once said that strength was not only always about triumphing against the odds, but it was also about supporting those in need, about standing up for people who cannot fend for themselves and about always getting back on your feet even when you do not know if you can make it.

Since the decease of my mother, I tried to estimate the ways and means in which our lives were influenced by her. Her love was the keel upon which her life was constructed. From it, we gained the courage to chase our passions, the steadfastness to overcome obstacles and the empathy to help others. She was a great mother and a very strong-willed and authoritative figure in the family. To date, her influence is felt in all the decisions we make and all the achievements we make in life.

To this day, her influence shows in all the choices we make and all the successes we celebrate in life. For my sisters, it was through her empowerment that they naturally became my mother because she is no longer with us. They always see to it that I am in the best of health, mind, and life, checking on me as always as she used to do. During the worst of times, they refuse to let me break and remind me of where we have come from and how far we still have to go. My sisters are just an extension of my mother, guiding, supporting, and ensuring that no matter what comes our way, we'll keep moving forward with the resilience she instilled in us.

Daya's story is a true testimony to comforting love; a love that changes rather than console. It has the power to replace what has been lost, to determine the destiny of her children, and to build for them, come what may. My mother was a silent and a strong woman and her love will always be with me, my sisters and all of us.

She was not only a mother but a warrior, a defender, and a mentor as well. And as much as she may no longer be here with us, I know her love and strength is with all of us.

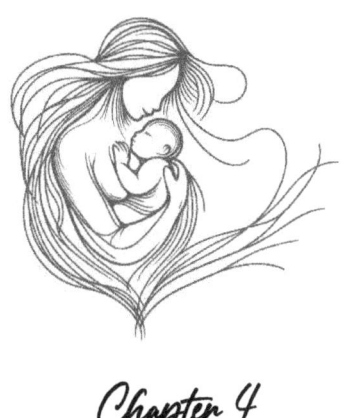

Chapter 4

Courage to Stand Alone

Courage is often misunderstood. It is not the lack of fear, and it cannot always be defined by great deeds and magnificent accomplishments. Real valour is not loud; instead, it is a firm and unwavering presence, especially when one has to act alone during critical moments. My mother Daya showed this courage several times in her lifetime. She did not budge from the choices she made and she did not yield to the pressure of family, society and sometimes even us, her children. Her decision to stand alone defines her life and ours, reminding us that the strength to make difficult choices emanates from within.

My mother's courage was her most defined character trait, and it shone even brighter when tragedy struck. My father, who was a government official, was met with an unexpected demise, leaving his wife and children stranded. In India when a government employee dies, the government offers a job to one of his family members as a compensation of sorts. This offer can get the family financial stability in a very short time and it was an offer my mom was expected to secure. However, this meant choosing who among the family members would go for this job. Daya had all the leeway; she could take up the job herself, or give it to me as her son, or even offer it to the eldest sister, Preeti. All the members of the family had their suggestions on what she should do. It was considered logical for people to choose a stable government job in such circumstances. However, my mother did not make any hasty decisions, even in the face of insurmountable uncertainty.

Daya was a forward-thinking woman and while she might not have been as literate as some people around her might have been, she possessed something better — knowledge and intuition. She realised that even though the offer seemed lucrative, it was going to be in our best interest not to take it. Rather than grabbing the opportunity to secure it for herself or imposing it on one of us, she opted to let my sister, Preeti, prepare and sit for her own government entrance examinations. Daya believed in hard work. Her reluctance to take up the job offer stemmed from her intolerance of easy fixes. And she was right. Preeti worked really hard to get herself a government job, and she got it on the basis of merit, not because it was presented to her on a silver platter.

Now, when I look back, I can only marvel at how much strength it required for my mother to stand by that decision. It wasn't an easy choice. The decision to turn down that job opportunity was met with considerable criticism from the rest of the family, and it would have been much easier just to accept it to help the family be financially secure right away. However, Daya was not interested in temporary fixes; she was interested in giving her children the best chance at success and the means to secure financial freedom in the long run. In this way, by allowing us to choose our own freedoms, she taught us the value of striving for what we wanted and not taking the easy way out. It is a lesson that defines the role we play in our own lives and the lives of those around us.

Daya's courage to stand alone was not only displayed on occasions that required a life-changing decision like this. It also manifested in the seemingly minor, more mundane decisions where she was the one to fight for what she ultimately knew was right, not just for us as a family, but also against what had potentially been culturally imposed upon her.

As a single mother raising two daughters in India, all my mother heard all the time was questions regarding the future of my sisters. Relatives, neighbours and acquaintances would inquire, "Who will marry them?" As though my father's absence meant that my sisters' prospect of securing suitable partners had dramatically decreased. The societal expectation from my mother was to concentrate more on finding good suitors for her daughters, as that was believed to make way for a secured future for women. But Daya did not look at things in the same way as the others. She never allowed society to decide the fate of her daughters.

"I'm not raising them to be dependent on anyone," she would state. "I'm raising them to be strong, independent women who can stand on their own. " This was a very progressive way of thinking in the society that valued a woman by how well she could wed. Though my mother was a woman of her word, the words people had for her did not matter to her. She was determined and would sooner fight for her daughters' education and freedom than to just marry them off. Because of her courage and strength, my sisters were able to make their own careers and be masters of their own lives.

One of the bravest episodes that I observed in my mother occured when I was in my final year studying engineering. We were deep in the throes of financial ruin, and my college fees were still due. It was a good sum of Rs. 20,000. We found ourselves in a position where we couldn't find the means to pay the fees.

In such a situation, the seemingly reasonable thing would be to seek assistance from other extended family members or friends, but my mother was a woman of principles and an unfaltering devotion to self-sufficiency. She had always stuck to the rule that we should not depend on anyone in our lives. This was one of those moments when it appeared that there was no other way round. Still, she was unwavering on her decision not to take a dime from anyone.

Then, a miracle happened. In her desperation to find a solution, my mother recalled that there was a bank account that was never used for many years. She asked me to see whether it still held some cash that could be retrieved, but neither of us had any expectations. I went to the bank, setting aside any hopes of getting anything out of it. But when I came back, I had tears in my eyes—it had Rs. 35,000 in it, more than enough to pay my fees. Whether it was a sheer stroke of luck or not, I do not know. But at that moment, it felt like nothing short of a miracle. That day, my mother taught me an invaluable lesson: sometimes, it might be far better to stand alone, to rely on nothing but one's own wits to come up with solutions; the payoff often was greater than one had ever dreamed of.

Her courage was not only in the financial aspect of her life; it included all the aspects of her life during the final year of my B. Tech, one day, I light-heartedly mentioned to my mother that some of my friends were planning to prepare for their MBA, and I also wanted to do it. While I categorically supported the idea, I was aware that it would cost a great deal of money. But as the forward-thinking woman that she was, my mother insisted that I should continue with it. "It will take time," she argued, "But the outcome will justify the efforts put into it."

This decision also meant bearing extra costs while getting loans and prolonging my opportunity to enter the labour force by two more years. While my mother's friends supported my desire to pursue an MBA, there were many who were sceptical. They told us that pursuing another degree was unwise because it did not generate income immediately. But my mother had a vision for the future of her son. Having faith in the fact the MBA would be an expansion of opportunities for me, she was equipped with the necessary courage to fight and make it happen, despite the sceptical points of view of some individuals.

Getting the loan to fund my MBA education was another time where her fearlessness was evident to me. At first my loan application was turned down by the bank because there was no earning member in our family. I returned home with my spirit dampened, wondering how we would cope with things. However, my mother was not willing to surrender. The very next day she went directly to the bank and demanded to speak to the manager of the bank. She was very confident in my abilities and let the manager know that despite financial difficulties she would find a way to help her son with his educational endeavour, but it would be foolish for the bank not to invest in the future and mind of an intelligent young man. She put forth her argument with such confidence and conviction that, at the end of the conversation the manager agreed to grant us a loan. She displayed an amazing power; a woman with no prior knowledge in finance, she was ready to defend her son and fight for what she thought was best for him. It was a powerful lesson in the importance of hard work and never giving up on oneself, which I have taken with me to this day.

My mother was a fearless woman who never displayed any indecisiveness. She stood by every decision she made, even the ones nobody else understood. Her bravery and deftness shone through, as much in the life-altering decisions as in her day-to-day choices. Her courage was not loud, demonstrated through monumental gestures. It was subtle and discreet. It showed in her determination to stay put, to swim against the tide, and in her unfathomable faith in us, her children. She never cared for societal acceptance. Instead, her decisions were always informed by a far-sightedness.

Humble and unassuming, Daya also demonstrated courage in embracing her weaknesses and flaws. Since she had never worked before, she had to adapt to handling household finances, dealing with paperwork, and making crucial decisions in areas ranging from education to health and law. Yet she had never backed down from these challenges. Instead, she confronted every challenge and relied on her own instincts to win it over.

In fact, fearlessness was not only demonstrated by my mother in taking individual decisions but also in moulding us to be individuals. She made us believe that we were strong enough to stand on our two feet without having to depend on someone or something else. We could do things our own way and come up with decisions that suited our abilities, and more to the point, we could do things independently. Inadvertently, in doing so, she had paved our paths to a good life with as much integrity as independence. My siblings and I cut from the same cloth, have carved out our own lives for ourselves without burdening anyone else with the responsibility.

As I look back, I begin to understand that my mother was not entirely fearless. Her courage lay in taking action despite all the fear. Her bravery lay in her ability to remain undeterred even in the face of great uncertainties. Her story is a testament to righteousness, the will to choose the right path, even when tempted to take the easy way out. It is about holding your moral ground, even when your vision is blurry, and the future seems bleak.

Daya's legacy of courage continues to guide me, my sisters, and all those who knew her. She showed us that sometimes, the bravest thing you can do is stand firm in your beliefs, even when the world around you is telling you to do otherwise.

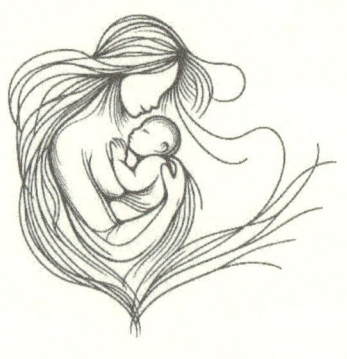

Chapter 5

The Journey to Financial Freedom

Financial freedom is more than having money in the bank to merely get by-it is an issue about personal dignity, freedom, and control over one's own destiny. In my mother Daya's case, this was not a question but a mandate after my father's tragic passing. With three young children to feed and raise on a shoestring budget, she had to take up the mantle of becoming the financial backbone of our family. But her fight to earn financial independence was not just a fight for survival but also a fight for the future of the children who longed to be provided with opportunities, stability, and pride.

When my father passed away, Daya was thrust into an unfamiliar role as the sole decision-maker in our house. Like many others of her generation, she had never managed the purse strings of a family in life; overnight, suddenly, it was all on her. Piling rice and vegetables on the table or paying the electricity bill would no longer do it. Instead, we were getting each penny to stretch as far as possible, setting aside enough for our education, never again feeling weighed down by those struggles, and we were so gruelling at every turn.

When consumed by that huge gulf of grief, she channeled all that pain into action and desire and purpose by channeling it further into a deep love for us, into a burning energy that made her want to ensure that we wouldn't miss the opportunities life had in store for us.

The first challenge she was to face was to manage this puny ₹5,000 per month pension left to her after my father's death. It was hardly enough for the family of four to survive. But my mother never let the scarcity make us feel deprived. She approached the situation with remarkable practicality, cutting back on expenses wherever possible. Meals became easier, but we never got hungry. Clothes were patched and mended, but we never went un-dressed. She became an expert in frugality, yet how she made sure that our lives never felt lacking in love, warmth, and hope.

One of the important lessons she taught me at the time was resourcefulness. Daya considered financial independence not only as bringing money into the home but also as being strategic and creative in what we had while being wise in decision-making. She could strategise on every purchase by considering long-term benefits as opposed to short-term comforts. It wasn't just to make it through the day; it was to ensure our tomorrow. The choices that she made at those moments would have paved the way for the economic security we would eventually enjoy.

We spent all our meagre income, but my mother's priority was always our education. I think she thought that once we were better educated, this cycle of deprivation would end, and we would be arming ourselves with skills to build a better life. No small matter what funding that education was, the fees for school mounted fast. Then came books and other expenses, and even at times, I felt it would not even be possible. Yet Daya never let us lose hope. She found ways to keep costs sometimes through sheer luck and often through her acumen in finance.

I remember very vividly one particular incident when my sister Preeti needed money to go to the coaching classes because she had to appear at competitive exams. The fees were steep and something we could never manage. But instead of giving up, she found a solution.

She contacted a shopkeeper in the locality, known to us, who would buy some of those handcrafted garments she had produced over the years. It is not a grand gesture, but it would suffice to pay the fees. Her readiness to do whatever was required, be it selling personal items or finding soft sources of income, was a testament to her resolve to never let our education fall victim to her decisions. But Daya's quest for financial independence was not just, in one way, a day-to-day survival strategy; it was also one of looking forward and sowing the seeds of stability over time. She understood that to be truly free, she had to ensure that we could stand on our own if need be, which also meant making difficult decisions such as not taking any loans from my family when we were really fighting to make ends meet.

It would have been easy to accept offers of help, but Daya was fiercely independent. She believed that relying on others for financial support would weaken our resolve and limit our ability to make our own choices.

Among so many moments, one of the most important events in the process of crystallising her financial philosophy was realising just how limited our financial deposits were. Life insurance was not something placed much importance on back then, and my father, like so many of his generation, did not foresee the need for substantial life insurance coverage. There was really very little leftover monetary value for the basic survival of our essential financial security and deposits that would need to be used for important life events, like education, weddings for my sisters, or emergencies that might befall us.

My mother never lagged in her efforts. She made it pretty clear at a young age how important it was to be financially independent. She didn't blow the situation off, being concerned or embarrassed about discussing our situation with us. She didn't sugarcoat what needed to happen in order for us to have security. She always believed that financial freedom was fundamental to personal dignity and family security. In belief of that principle, she shaped the ways we handled our circumstances.

My elder sister, Preeti, was the most responsible among the three of us and would step up when the family needed her to. With a crystal clear sense of duty, Preeti started maths tuitions, teaching those small kids living in our neighbourhood. Her commitment and talent as a teacher were so good that most of the children whom she taught passed their exams with glittering marks, achieving excellent grades and, consequently, pride in the parents. Preeti soon became very popular in the locality, and they knew that no matter how complex the mathematical problem was, it would be explained to the student in a way that even the weakest would feel comfortable understanding it.

Preeti started the day early, looking to herself for her own education and studies; by the afternoon, she was teaching 15 children from the neighbourhood and working until late at night. In the process, she was contributing to the purse of the family but, more importantly, becoming financially independent at an age that is impressively young. During many months of my graduation, she kept sending me money for my studies. Preeti was generous, hardworking, and had a big heart, and her help became a lifeline for me during those months. She sacrificed so much in order to help us all move forward; I never forgot that.

My mother, Daya, never hesitated to use our savings and deposits for our education. She believed that education was the future for us and was always of the notion that any investment in learning would reap much more returns than any savings we could bank. She strongly felt that once we were successful in our chosen fields, we would one day earn much more than the small savings at the time. And so, whenever it was time to pay school fees or finance our studies, my mother would never regard that money as a loss but as an investment in our potential.

Actually, my mother always had in mind that we should never afford to lose a chance to invest in education simply because of a lack of money. She often said, "If you are capable, there will always be a way." The forward-thinking philosophy she designed inspired us to push ourselves while knowing she believed in our ability to get the most out of every educational opportunity we had. It was this belief in us that powerfully enabled all three of us to try hard for success and to achieve financial independence from an early stage of our lives.

My sister Priya, who was much younger than me, was equally active in making sure our family did not falter. She used to take great care to see if I had everything necessary to study properly; sometimes, she had even taken out some responsibilities way over her age. All three of us carried on this burden because my mother's philosophy had driven us forward. She explained to us that financial independence was not about the money in our bank account but it rather meant having the freedom to make choices, the power to support one another; and the ability to take care of our own future.

However, the process of attaining financial independence was tough and an emotional experience for me. There have been moments when financial constraints seemed overwhelming; however, it is because my mother believes in the power of education and financial independence that we did not get derailed. She was practical, yes, but she was also profoundly optimistic about what we could achieve if we stayed focused. Her belief in long-term gain compared to short-term sacrifice made all the difference. She never made us feel inferior due to our financial status; instead, she always inspired us to grow above this thing, work hard, and create opportunities for ourselves.

Finally, about more than just managing money, this approach to Daya's financial freedom was teaching resilience, responsibility, and independence. She taught us that security came not from holding onto what you have but from having confidence in believing that you could do things well and investing in the future with gladness in your heart. This lesson has guided us up until now and still shapes our decisions and successes. She not only established her financial independence but instilled it in us; she made sure we could walk confidently in this world, knowing that we had the tools and the mindset to create our own.

Through these years, Daya's unwavering determination never ceased to amaze me. She not only managed to keep us afloat but also found ways to build a financial foundation that would later allow us to thrive. She taught me the importance of planning for the future, no matter how uncertain the present seemed. She was of the nature type, and she felt that this moment in time needed to be looked beyond, and some decisions were made for our betterment in the long term. She would always stay ahead of the curve when I couldn't even see it; she ensured that we would have those opportunities to succeed even though things were bleak at the time.

Her ability to manage our finances, even when this resource was in such limited supply, eventually paid out in ways we could neither have imagined nor have conceived of. The more we grew up and matured into successful careers, the less we faced financial hardship during those early years of our lives. But I will never forget how, no matter what was going on, Daya always kept her eye on the bigger picture.

She wasn't just focused on surviving the moment—she was building a future for us, one small step at a time.

To me, the process of becoming financially independent of the same mother is her refusal to perceive what was done to us as who we are. My mother could have stayed content that whatever was done to us would stick to determine our destiny.

Instead, she fought to construct an alternate story about our family, a story in which to overcome some of the obstacles standing in our way and secure a more promising future. Her strength, resourcefulness, and the unshakeable conviction that financial independence was a power setting the tone for everything that followed. What makes her story is not so much one of survival but one of empowerment. She didn't just keep us afloat; she equipped and armed us to be achievers in the long haul.

I still remember the day I got my first salary. I rang her and said, "What can I get for you? At the end of the day, all I have is all because of you." My mom was crying, and what she said next I didn't expect. She said,

"Go to a nearby temple or an orphanage and make some donations. Help those who need support.".

I was taken aback. After all the financial hardship my family had been through, I had considered that she would suggest putting some money into savings or perhaps buying herself some gold or new clothes— things she had not indulged in for so long. Instead, her first instinct was to ask me to give from my first salary, to donate and help those less fortunate. I could not believe it.

She continued, "Remember, you survived with limited resources, and the way you're going, you'll continue earning much more in the future. But always remember: the more you empower others and support the needy, the universe will give you much more than what you donate."

At that moment, her words struck me very deep. Having just received my first salary, and after all those years of financial struggle, this certainly wasn't what I needed to hear. But this was typical Daya—all thinking beyond immediate gains, seeing the bigger picture. She embodied a sense of empowerment in everything she did, and this was no different. In that instance, she taught me an important lesson on how giving works, reminding me that the base of financial independence is not to reap personal fruits but to use what is available to uplift others.

Here, her philosophy of giving doesn't stop with financial independence but spreads across all aspects of life. She truly believed that real success is not the amount you earn but how much you give back to the world. So, she not only ushered us into financial stability and also made sure we were well aware of giving back and sharing stability with others. Empowerment to her was far more than just securing financial stability-it was to let one understand his or her responsibility which came with such empowerment.

Daya's financial independence was independent in more ways than she could possibly know. She and her financial power allowed us, her children, to do things on our own terms. This stuff about financial security isn't just about your money in the bank; it's about being sure in the pursuit of your dreams, with risks and standing on your own two feet. It is about ownership of life. Even when the world around you seems to be crumbling, such confidence gives one a feeling of being in control. Ultimately, it was my mother's desire for economic independence, which was more than a struggle just to get by; it also was a hope to have a foundation to construct our own lives. That is, we would be in an excellent position to pursue all our dreams and never fear the possibility of failure: we have resourcefulness as well as a support system to achieve success.

But that was more than practical; it was an act of deep love, for she truly believed that economic independence was transformative and would give life its first chance to find stability. Daya's legacy continues to be that of strength, resourcefulness, and determination. Being illiterate with no formal education, I was baffled all the time how this lady could possibly have developed that thinking process. She once told me, "If you are good and resourceful, then money follows." For her, having the confidence to start at nothing and to build something incredible was resourcefulness. She believed that money does matter, but it merely serves as a tool and not as the end.

There was a sense of fearlessness about the way she handled her finances-never fearing to put everything on the line for our future. She invested all the money and financial securities in our education, confident that this was the best way to secure not just our future but the confidence we needed to pursue our dreams. "What am I supposed to do with this money," she would say, "if I can't even give you the confidence, the education, and the support to get these things you want?" That fearlessness, that willingness to take risks for the sake of her children's success, is what really defined her approach to financial freedom.

She knew in the end, the greatest investment she could make was in us. Her example teaches us that financial independence is not just about survival; it's more important to thrive. We find ourselves in a life where we have the confidence to make decisions free from the shackles of financial insecurity. Her journey continues to inspire me, reminding me that financial stability is not a goal but the very basis for living a life filled with dignity, peace, and freedom to achieve your dreams.

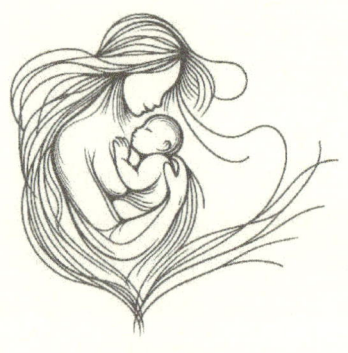

Chapter 6

Optimism Delivers Success

Optimism is not ignorance about the adversities; on the contrary, optimism identifies the adversities and faces them without letting them control. Optimism, in its most raw sense, is the notion that no matter how bad it gets, someday it will get better. It is an attitude that propels you toward the next step, even if it looks like the whole world is caving in on you. Indeed, my mother, Daya, was a perfect example: she embodied this philosophy. To her, optimism was not just a state of mind that could fade so easily; it was a way of life. It is this hope that helped her get through some of the most difficult and painful periods in her life and, thus, helped form the lives of her children. Her optimism did not just bring hope but also results.

For as long as I can remember, my siblings and I understood that our mother saw life differently than other people. She was one who never feared challenges; she took them head-on with full force. She had faced death when my father died when I was a child, and she was left to fend for three young children. And many would have thought that she would have broken under the pressure. But not Daya. She did not pay much attention to the past or what was said by other people but to what lay ahead. She wouldn't allow herself and her children to get buried in sorrow. Her optimism was not a denial of the fact that times were hard; it was the faith that even in the face of disaster, there would be a way.

Of all the times when I mentioned how my mother's optimism defined our lives, I remember the day when I got the first offer for employment with Tata Consultancy Services. It was nearly ten at night when they issued the final list, when zero-day campus placements were happening- an event very crucial for me and other students who had invested a lot of effort and time in building their careers. I was drowned in joy seeing my name among the selected few. The first person I told this to, of course, was my mother.

I never knew what she thought when I told her the news by looking at her face. She kept silent for a good five minutes. Then we both cried—cried tears of joy, tears of relief, and most of all, tears of gratitude. It was more than taking up a job; it represented something. She had been with me for six years, waited, believed in me, encouraged me, and fought for me. Indeed, that belief was made to ring true. "I knew this day would come," she said, her voice so calm that a person would hardly notice the rush of emotions. "I always knew that you would make it.

It captures my mother in a nutshell and depicts who she was in one moment. She did not need to think twice to believe what she had been told because she knew much regarding the fruits of hard work and perseverance. Her optimism was not just hopefulness; it was based on the belief that tenacity and faithfulness would eventually pay dividends in success. This was belief that had seen us through the darkest hours of our family and now, the fruits were ripe to be reaped.

But that day was just the start of it all. A few years later, my sister Preeti also claimed her moment of triumph. She had spent months of dedicated hard work and preparation to crack the Staff Selection Commission (SSC) examinations and emerged victorious by acquiring a government job. She felt at one point that the world was conspiring against her due to the cut-throat competition, but still, she continued. But Mum never lost hope in Preeti and was very confident that she would clear the examination, which is what she had been doing always.

As if she was trying to be placating, she used to tell Preeti, who doubted her ability after some failure: "You have done all the hard work already. It's only a matter of time now." And that's what was actually true. I never could have thought that Preeti had done much work for this success, and our mother was always supportive of her. It was not a passive kind of optimism that my mother had; it was an active one. She did not wait and expect everything to turn out all right. She encouraged and reassured us, bolstered our self-esteem, and urged us forward when the hurdles seemed insurmountable.

My younger sister, Priya, also acted exactly the same way. She pursued her course in engineering, a course known to be competitive and not very friendly to female students in our society back then. There were times when Priya felt pressure coming from her academic challenges, but, as usual, my mother was her star of hope. "You are stronger than you think you are," she would counsel Priya. "So, you just have to persist, and at some point, things will work out."

And, of course, my mother - how am I going to utter those words? Again, she proved right. Priya managed to settle for her job and, later on, established herself as a professional in a French consulting company. Today, she is well-established, doing a great job in her career, and her confidence never falters. Our optimism and our existence have been founded on the faith and confidence that my mother had in us. It was nothing more simplistic than looking at a half-full glass, but rather, the opposite constantly filled her glass, day by day, hour by hour. She is persevering and unyielding in hope.

My journey wasn't over yet; my mother's optimistic attitude greatly influenced me. For half the year, I was working at Tata Consultancy Services when, one day, my luck struck in the form of a transfer to London. There definitely began a new chapter in my life, full of opportunities and new hurdles. Emigrating and starting anew elsewhere could have been very daunting. Still, my mother's voice kept ringing in my head each time.

"You have come this far," she used to tell me whenever I questioned my capabilities. "Now, the sky is the limit.".

The encouragement she gave me helped me approach the change with lots of confidence and, for that reason, commit fully to the opportunity. The transfer to London was not just up the ladder of career advancement; it was the realization of my mother's faith in me. For that moment and thereafter, I grasped onto her optimism and never at any time had a moment of doubt in anything that all else will be well despite how bad things are.

Yet another brilliant example of how my mother's optimism used to influence us is when I repaid my education loan back. After considering all that was on offer for an MBA program, I decided to take a seven-year loan which entailed its own series of opportunities as well as risks offered on the table. It had taken a lot of effort to get this loan in the first place, and there were moments when I was questioning whether I was capable of taking on this type of commitment for such a long period. But my mother was never unsure of me for even a single moment in my life.

Every time I posed the question to her on how this repayment was even possible, she'd just smile and say that "We'll find a way." "You will repay it much sooner than you imagine".

That I could clear the loan as well, and that too, within six months was a surprise in itself. What would have normally taken seven long years was completed in half a year. It was a moment of immense pride not only for me but also for my loved ones. My mother was not left shaken up by that though. All her life she has always known that I would be able to complete this feat.

The bank manager, who originally denied and subsequently approved my loan, still relishes telling to this day how a seven-year loan was paid back in six months. He himself identifies me as an example of what determination and opportuneness can lead to, but it was really my mother's optimism that delivered that success. Her belief in me couldn't have been stronger, and that is exactly what made me go further than I ever believed I could.

As days passed, outcomes of our toil started to reveal themselves slowly. Gradually we began to come out of our problems, and it seemed as if even time was turning in our favor. Finally, the years of hardship and turmoil, compromise, and waiting for better times ahead were coming to an end. And all this my mother, an optimist, that force that did not let us lose under whatever circumstance.

But, amazingly, my mom's optimism wasn't just rejoicing with victories that arrived. In fact, it was all about embracing the positive outlook of life even when things did not go according to plan. There were quite a number of times when life took quite unexpected turns, when journeys seemed blurry, or when adversities hit, yet my mom never lost the ability to look for the positive in anything given.

This too shall pass," she would remind us during some of the hardest periods that life could offer. "There will always be better days."

Such a perspective on even the most complex situations served as our hope to continue. She did not dismiss the struggles we had. However, she was not going to let those define us either. She made it a norm to reverse the roles of success and failure and to treat every failure as temporary and every challenge as a learning point. She made us understand that optimism does not mean being blind to the problems around us. Rather it means hope in improvement and striving towards that light with hope.

Perhaps the impact which my mother's optimism brought in me was related to education. When I declared my will for pursuing the MBA degree, I was pretty much aware of how expensive it would be to my family. It was costly and sitting with a loan for seven years sounded scary. She didn't even think twice about that decision.

'You must do it,' she said. "It will be a sound investment that will begin to bring fruits even before you know it."

Only rarely would she doubt the decision we had made to continue our education despite the fact that sometimes, even to us, that decision seemed to raise doubts about its soundness. Some people frowned at it, saying that I had no business going for higher education since I needed to get some immediate source of income, but it was my mother who anticipated the future, long term as opposed to catering for the immediate present. She knew that what we underwent today would pay off tomorrow, and she had her unwavering hope to support that conviction, even when everybody else around me disapproved of it.

It is only now that I understand that hope is the greatest legacy my mother had bequeathed on all of us. It was not so much the good outlook in life; it was the fight of trying to overcome the challenges of life knowing that the situation would improve. She epitomized hope as she always looked on the brighter side and encouraged us to try as much as we could even when the going got tough.

Actually, it is the story of optimism and hope, something that makes one believe that in whatever situation, there is always a bit of hope. This does not mean turning a blind eye to life's challenges but instead deciding to focus on one's opportunities amidst the mountain of challenges ahead. The confidence she had that things could be better was making her stay strong, making us all stronger and prompting us to keep going forward even when we did not quite know where we were headed. And finally, her optimism paid off in ways other than career success. It wrote the script of our lives, for which parts may today serve as inspiration to the readers.

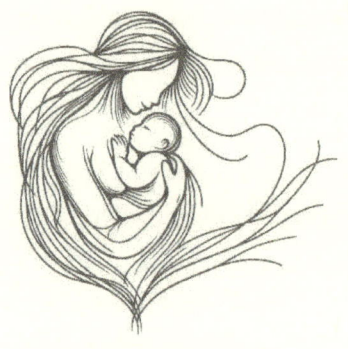

Chapter 7

Finding Happiness in Small Moments

Most people find happiness in major gestures or historic feats, but to me and several others, happiness is much more. Such a person was my mother, Daya, for whom happiness was never a question of material things or expensive experiences but rather the mere thread of daily life. She could find light in the darkness, the small victories and quiet pleasures we so often miss. This philosophy led to not only her but also our lives, teaching us the profound lesson that happiness can always be found, even amidst hardship.

2011 to 2015 is a very significant chapter of our family's life. It was the time of glee and transition the outgoing to the new beginning all her children one by one started their married lives. Those achievements in the lives of children constitute celebration moments for most parents, but my mom also made it a time when her mothering instincts and deep involvement in our lives came into play. She was very keen on our going out and finding our appropriate mates, but she was equally keen on marrying us off to families with values aligned with ours and people who would encourage and support our development. She had an uncanny instinct about what was good for us when we did not even see it.

One of those traits we admired and sometimes were afraid of her for. My mother never sat back to watch; she was all involved, advising us at times and, at times, even making decisions for us. All this, however, was preceded by her excess love for us and true concern for our happiness. She didn't find happiness in the control of the outcome nor did she know that we were alone building sound, supporting lives for ourselves. As I look back on those marriage preparation years, I can vividly see the smile in her eyes- not just during the happenings themselves but for the relationships being forged.

She delighted in seeing how the lives of her children flourished and how our family kept growing and becoming more meaningful and loving. Whether it was choosing the perfect sari to be worn during which ceremony, finalising the minute particulars of the ceremonies, or deciding which caterer to use and which decorators, my mother thought herself pleased with all the minute and finest details of each wedding. She savoured every aspect, enjoyed every step, and was proud to ensure that it all went along flawlessly- all this without compromising her deep conviction of putting family first. Yet, there was always this quiet part of her which secretly yearned for a moment of peace time when she could put away all responsibilities and untie the tension knots in her neck.

After years of family being first, it was in 2015 that my mother finally granted herself the sinecure of well-deserved break when she decided to visit Kashmir, the place she had long yearned to see. She was doing something entirely for herself the first time in years, and the excitement among her family circle before the journey was palpable. For weeks, nothing else was spoken of.

She sat with a gleam in her eyes, planning what she might take with her and imagining the mountain air. For someone who had spent all her life other-focused, this trip was a selfish act of self-care; it brought her a kind of joy that we hardly saw in her. It was not about reaching some destination, after all; it was about freedom - a chance for her to step out of her daily responsibilities and concentrate on being happy. When she returned from Kashmir, she was bubbling with excitement.

She would talk day and night about the mountains with a sheet of snow on top, the crisp, clean air, and the sweet kindness of the people of Kashmir. The way she described houseboats on Dal Lake, the full-on markets, and the beauty of it all made it crystal clear that this particular trip was life-changing for her. She had been taken away, even if only for a little while, into a world that was soothing and peaceful, a world a thousand miles removed from the daily grind she carried around with her for years. What was incredible about her experience was not the grandeur of the trip she was on but rather the manner in which she delighted in the simple moments.

She talked little of luxury rooms and costly food. She rather enjoyed quiet conversations with small locals about the beauty of a well-woven shawl and the fresh taste of Kashmiri tea. She was satisfied most in these small encounters. The stories were not about great adventures but were about people, moments of small kindness and beauty which characterised her journey. My mother wasn't visiting Kashmir to enjoy a holiday. She needed to take a break so that she could remind herself that after all the years, she could still be happy for herself.

She was breathing freely, as if the weight of decades had rolled off her shoulders and finally, for the first time since the rigid responsibilities she led consumed her life, it all settled atop her shoulders as she lifted responsibility. And while that was a rare respite from her frugal self, it was far from the first time she had enjoyed life in such minuscule details.

Daya often found ways to seek joy in simple everyday moments. Among the greatest pleasures, she took in life was sitting on our porch with a cup of tea late in the afternoons and watching the world go by. To an outsider, it may look like an ordinary activity, but for her, it was a moment of quiet reflection, a time for her to take stock of her day and appreciate the simple beauty of life. And it was in the quiet of the stillness that she would call us over to share the moments with her and discuss our day. No urgency to anything, no task in hand, just a shared cup of tea and a few words and comfort in the silence of it all. It was in those tiny moments of human connection that did her fuel. The second source of glee for my mother was her garden.

Our home wasn't big, but she had a small patch of land which mostly consisted of flowers and herbs. She loved to see them grow and bloom; it was her favourite hobby. She knelt in the dirt, tending her garden with almost the same amount of care and attention to detail she had for everything else in life, and felt that those flowers symbolised hope, resilience, and cycles of life. Even at her worst moments, she could soothe herself in her garden - always knowing that something beautiful would bloom in time, as long as there was care and enough patience. She even grew proud in her old age of the growing independence of her children after the Kashmir trip.

Each time one of us marked a new milestone in their career or personal life, she would celebrate it not with fanfare but with quiet pride. These weren't the ostentatious parties that some parents might throw them- they were intimate moments where she would offer just the right word or subtle smile, satisfied that her own sacrifices had gotten us to where we were. When her health began to decline, she was still as full of joy over the simple things as ever.

Although she knew at times what was wrong with her, she never lost that zest for life's simplest things: the strokes of a soft breeze, a visit from an old friend, or a meal shared with her family. She never lost that joyful laugh, her appreciation for all her life built. Daya was a simple philosophy in words but profound in its nature: life is fleeting, and real happiness does not come from what one achieves but from how one lives each day.

She taught us the nature of joy. It doesn't have to be sought after in far-off places or grand accomplishments. It is right there, from the moments we spend with loved ones to the beauty of the sunrise or even in the taste of a good cup of tea, for it lies happiness in this is in being present to appreciate life in all its imperfections. In a world of continuous striving for more, my mother taught us that true fulfilment emanates from appreciating what is. Simple, grateful, and joyful is the byproduct of her legacy: a reminder that even in the greatest challenges of life, light can always be found if one's eyes are open to look for it.

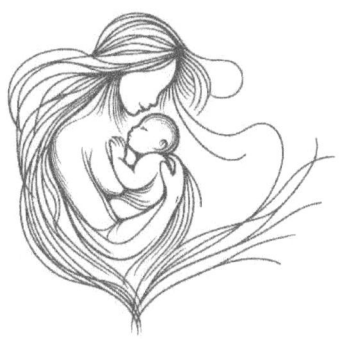

Chapter 8

Curiosity for Lifelong Learning

C uriosity never fades with age; it merely deepens as the world becomes a place where every experience holds a lesson. My mother, Daya, was no exception. Her curiosity was the driving force behind her lifelong love of learning. It kept her mind sharp and her spirit young. She didn't stop growing just because her formal education was over or because life became difficult. Instead, she embraced new experiences, sought out knowledge in the most unlikely of places, and seized every chance to broaden her understanding of the world around her. It mattered little where she was or what she already knew; she was always eager to know more.

One of the best examples of her boundless curiosity and love for learning came in 2018 when she finally obtained her family visitor visa for the UK. She was refused entry twice, but two rejections didn't stop her resolve to visit the UK and explore life in London for which she had only heard stories and images. Each rejection was a knock, but not enough to keep my mum's spirit down. For her, every setback was only a temporary obstruction, not a permanent barrier. She applied again with even more determination, and the excitement when the visa arrived was matchless.

Visiting the UK was a monumental experience for her. This was her first journey out of India, where she had spent all her life. The thought of going to a foreign land with its different languages, customs, and culture really thrilled her more than intimidated her. Unlike many who might feel apprehensive about venturing into unknown territory, my mom embraced it as an opportunity for learning. "Life is too short not to explore," she said before her trip. "Every new place, every new person has something to teach us.".

It was as if the whole world had opened its eyes and looked inside with great curiosity when she reached London. Everything was new to her: dresses and ways people spoke about things, the streets, the architecture, and naturally enough, even the weather. The fast pace of London, historical landmarks, and diversity captured her. Grand sights interested her, but everyday life rivalled it. She was no tourist; she had become a student of life, absorbing everything around her with a sense of wonder you would expect from a child seeing the world for the first time.

Her first experience in the UK set the tone for the rest of her trip. When she landed at Heathrow Airport, she seemed lost. The grandness of the airport and her limited knowledge of the English language proved to be a great challenge for her to navigate through to the arrivals area. But instead of panicking, she sought help, this time around coming in the form of a Pakistani pilot who had noticed her confusion. Being aware that she was not very conversational in the English language, he switched to Urdu, even speaking to her with kindness and respect, and took her quietly to the arrival section where I was waiting for her.

As she waited to send me off at the airport, she never stopped talking about the episode. Her face was all aglow while recounting how respectful and helpful the pilot had been. "He was so kind," she said, her voice full of gratitude. "In India, we hear so many negative things about Pakistan and their people, but here I was, helped by a Pakistani man in a foreign land. We are all the same at heart, no matter where we come from."

That experience marked her. She wasn't only looking for her way through the airport; it was breaking down and unravelling everything that had been passed on to her as tradition, everything that she'd been given to believe. The world had always intrigued her, but at that point, she found that knowledge is also unlearning; it takes away a certain number of preconceived notions of the kind to embrace the humanity of a stranger, whatever the colour or system that has been built around them. This lesson she took back with her and would sometimes speak of it. And it reminded her that at the heart of humanity lies beyond borders.

Once seated in London, she wouldn't rest on her laurels. New discoveries were made daily, and she enjoyed them to the fullest. She was most struck by the level of respect people accorded one another, irrespective of gender, race, or nationality. There, she had seen in the city of India how such family expectations burden those who should be free, but here in London, she saw that culture put great importance on equality, which she had never known anywhere else. She marvelled at how women were treated with respect, as they walked with power, and their free movement unencumbered by the bonds that bound them so oft elsewhere in this world.

What I love about this place, she said to me one evening during her visit, is the sense of equality. Here, people respect each other, whoever they are. It does not matter where you come from or who you are-they treat you with the same respect.

This opened her eyes and made her realise that respect and dignity are not only basic rights but also are not bound by anyone's background or gender. The profound admiration for the British culture taught her something she already knew- treating people with kindness and respect to see it practised in a different country reinforced this belief within her.

Despite her lack of knowledge of the English language, my mother still wanted to venture out into the city of London alone. She wanted to see things for herself, but on her own terms and without any assistance, and no one, not even the rather confusing use of the English language, was going to stop her. I remember well when she came to me and asked for £50. She had given it considerable thought that she wanted to go shopping all by herself, without any assistance from me. First, she approached me hesitantly. You don't know English that well," I said to her. "I will bring you everything you need." But she insisted.

"You never stop learning in life," she said, her voice firm with conviction. "When you are stuck, do not be afraid of asking for help. Interact with people— whether they are strangers or old friends. You learn so much by talking to other people. Different angles, new input. That is how you grow."

She was very determined. Here she was, in a foreign country, not even able to say more than a few words in the local language and still unwilling to depend on others. She wanted to explore the city by herself, learn from this experience, and show herself that she would be able to do it. With her £50 in hand and a sense of adventure in her heart, she set off on her solo journey.

When she came back in the afternoon, she beamed with joy. She had travelled alone on the streets, tried to communicate with the shopkeepers by hand gestures and some broken English phrases, and bought what was required. It was just a small victory, but for her, it meant much more; it marked the time that she remembered how curiosity and a will to learn can conquer whatever disability there may be. It was not that excitement over what she had purchased but the feeling of independence and success she had. She had tested her limits by stepping out of her comfort zone and came out successful.

Her query was not limited to the thrill of a shopping spree or a day of sightseeing. Every individual she met on the streets of London - a bus driver, a shopkeeper, or some passersby - was a school and an opportunity for learning on her part. She inquired, interacted with people and soaked in their stories. Fascinated by the diversity of the city, how people from every corner of the world were staying, working together, and existed harmoniously, marveling at an efficient system of public transportation, the streets kept clean, and respect for a public space.

One of her favourite pastimes during this trip was sitting in one of London's many parks and watching the world go by. She would find a bench and sit amidst the greenery, observe the people around her, see families having picnics, children playing, and couples walking hand in hand. It was all so different for her, yet she reveled in it. These quiet moments of observation proved to be very valuable for any form of education. It is the way people are living, their interaction with one another, and how different cultures can live peacefully.

Her last trip to the UK was also fulfilled in 2019. She was already confident in navigating the city by herself. She was very proud, moving around the entire city of London proudly, even though her English hadn't changed much. That did not bother her; the important thing was that she had learned, grown, and pushed herself. London was more than just a point of interest; it was an expansion of her perception and enjoyment of the quality of learning through others.

Daya's curiosity was not something limited to her travels. It may have been a thread throughout her life. She attacked everything from a new recipe to a master skill with exactly the same open-minded eagerness to learn. She was always hungry to learn a new recipe, mastering a new skill, simply learning from the people she was going to meet. She believed that life was full of lessons and that we had to find them.

My mother constantly reminded me, by example, that no one is ever too old to learn. Growth wasn't something I had learned would have occurred inside a classroom or when I was young; growth extends through the length of one's life as long as a person is open to it. It was that desire to learn that kept my mother young at heart and a willingness to experience new things that kept her spirit alive.

She was, in the sense of curiosity and exploration and lifelong passion for knowledge, a legacy. She proved to me that regardless of where we are in life, there is something always to find anew, something in which a lesson could be gained. She made me realise that staying curious would mean staying hooked into this world, to others, and to ourselves.

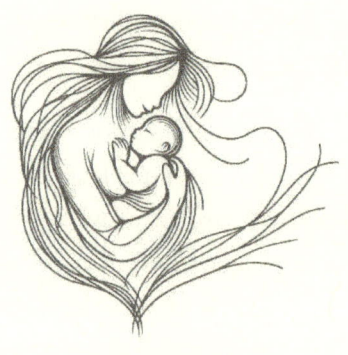

Chapter 9

Rooted in Cultural Heritage and Identity

For my mother, Daya, the cultural past was always something she was at least more or less fully immersed in. Above all, she would say that the most important thing is to stay close to where you come from: our traditions, our values, and our community. For her, heritage was not something you could set aside along life's journey; rather, it was the foundation on which everything rested. It defines who we are and, through that definition, is the reason for most of life's big choices. It gave her strength, clarity, and the deepest sense of belonging, and she passed all of it down to each one of us.

Another pillar of strength was her sister-in-law, my father's elder brother's wife, whom we affectionately called Amma. They never ever had disputes in their relationship. In different instances, they would not see others' points. My mother would sometimes criticise Amma openly and raise her grievances with her candid way of speaking. Amma would never reply back; she always remained cool and heard my mother patiently. Ultimately, however sharp the debate was, my mother would never go against Amma's discretion. She would agree to what Amma decided because she knew that whatever Amma would say was done for the good of the family through her judgment and sense of experience.

Such was the depth of her respect for her elders. She often used to tell us, "It is your Amma who set the culture of our family; everyone is so connected and attached to each other." The children of Amma treated my mother as if she were their own mother, though my mother, feeling her children's busy lives, kept her from doing much more for them than she wished. At the time my mother married into the family, Amma had been a mentor to her, familiarizing her with an entirely new world of married life and educating her in the customs and values of the family, which would define her place within the household. She made sure she would keep up all the values that had been taught throughout her lifetime. She was always so much in respect and harmony with the family, as well as in how she carried out her activities in all the spaces, whether at home or even at the workplace. These values were of a guiding principle for us, her children, as well.

When I got married, my mother's influence reached far and wide. We had the marriage in our ancestral village in Gonda, keeping up with the traditions. I invited 12 colleagues from London - foreigners who had worked with me and to my surprise and delight, every one of them attended the wedding. For them, it was an experience of a lifetime; they got to witness firsthand the effervescent three-day celebrations that filled their souls with joy and invigorated their senses as they inhaled an atmosphere dripping in the fragrance of fun-filled music, rituals, and festivities that were so different than anything they had known.

But what they cherished the most was not the grandeur of the event but the warmth and feeling of belonging in our village. They showed great respect towards us for choosing to solemnise the marriage in our ancestral home rather than having a more modern celebration in a cosmopolitan city or five-star hotel. For most of them, India has been a place of luxury hotels and big cities Weddings gave them an idea of real India, family, tradition, and value, so much at the core of every activity for many. My mother often referred to this event to remind people to motivate our family and others to stay connected with their roots and ancestral homes. "It is only in staying close to where we come from that we understand who we are," she would say.

In the latter half of my life, my mother often shifted her base to our ancestors' village. She would periodically visit to celebrate family occasions, like spending Diwali with her elder brother or participating in pooja ceremonies. She made it a ritual to attend the birthday celebrations of Bade Papa to the fullest so that she is present at every significant family gathering. These were no ordinary trips, but they were about staying low, drawing strength from what was familiar, and being in touch with values that had moulded her life. Being close to the roots was not just comforting for her but was the guiding light.

Her contact with our ancestral village and the family's cultural roots was far beyond nostalgia; it gave her a purpose. As life took her in different directions, she was never away from those places and the people who gave her her identity. It is there that, amidst familiar surroundings, she found clarity and direction to deal with the issues of life. Just as she drew strength from her heritage, she made sure we knew how important it was. She instilled within us a sense of respect for elders, a love for traditions, and a very deep sense of responsibility to remain connected with our roots, regardless of where life may lead.

Her philosophy of remaining close to the roots was not restricted to just family gatherings or festivals. It was the fabric of life sewn into the day-by-day. She made us believe that no matter how far we would travel, no matter how successful we would become, her heritage would always be there to help us navigate and guide us in making decisions, and to keep us grounded. "Roots aren't just where you come from," she said, "they're the foundation you stand on."

Reflecting on her life, I understand how deep her roots were, not just to her but also to all of us. Her connection to our family, culture, and community gave her the strength to lead, care for, and give a future life to her children in value. She held out with the wisdom of old times when modernity rushed us forward into a future that would, without her guidance, have shaken our sense of what really mattered. And in this, she freed us to understand who we are, where we are coming from, and what we stand for.

Mom stayed in a village. She stayed in a big extended family. So, if I had to say anything, it is with them that her identity would be defined. It was the place she grew up in some place, home no matter where life took us, and this place we lived lay much deeper there, hurt, time, and need. As our children grew up and began our separate lives, it would have been more than easy to lose track of our ancestral home and the traditions and people that had formed our past. Daya never did this, though-for her, keeping up with our village and our wider family was a first priority; she made sure we did too.

There is that saying she would say so often: "When you're lost in the world, lean into your roots." To my mother, that wasn't just something to say; it was how she lived. When hard choices loomed or when uncertainty threatened to asphyxiate, she sat still, thinking through things her culture, upbringing, and traditions in our little village had learned and shared with her. She always believed that the roots held every answer to questions in this world. A good sense of life, defined by generations telling us what lifestyle we held, guided her through every challenge in life.

The cultural practices and traditions she followed all her life were one way to bond with her roots. She would never let the importance of these rituals fade out of her mind, no matter how hectic life becomes or how much the world around us changes. One bright memory I have is of the festival celebrations every year in the village.

My mother made sure that we rejoiced in the celebrations with as much passion and respect that she had when she was young. Bright colors, traditions foods, prayers, and fully-recovery family reunions all etched what our origin was. It was time where happiness was being expressed but much more than anything Else. How we remain connected to culture.

My mother draws much power from her roots, even in bad times. I think of one of the toughest times that our family went through because we completely drained ourselves financially following the loss of my dad. At one point, everything wasn't quite so sure and a little frightening to read about for the future. However, it is there that Daya ran from everything else that was uncertain even the very traditions of our village. She reminded us often of how hard our foreparents were, the people who had to go through so many tribulations that were more heavy-duty than any of us ever did and endured. Their stories kept her and us strong. She'd say to us, "We come from a long line of strong, resilient people. Whatever we face, we will get through it, just like they did." And she was right. Her belief in our deep roots made it possible for us to move ahead in circumstances that seemed impossible at that moment.

One of the ways by which my mother has remained quite well connected to the cultural roots is how each of the marriages of her children is conducted in the village. It's one of those conscious decisions, and for which came a strong connection to our home and family along with traditions. Marriages in our cultures are far more than something that can bind two people together. But a communal celebration, with the whole village acting as a witness and giving a new beginning its blessing. It was during this time that my mother said everything which put together history, and the people who constituted a village were part of us, and we should respect that kind of bond at such an important time in our lives.

So, pretty big doohickeys of tradition and laughter would precipitate the wedding, with the family not alone but extended family and, indeed, much of the community at large; I can recall how my mother would beam with pride as she decided to conduct the ceremonies in our ancestral home, careful that every bit of this wedding is steeped in tradition- from rituals to food to music. It was not only the rituals; it was the feeling of belonging attached to it. It was more than a personal choice; it reminded us that our roots would always be with us, no matter where we travelled or how much we achieved. In some ways, it reminded us that we belonged to something more significant than ourselves and connected us to the generations before and probably after us into the future.

It wasn't a place for mere celebration but a refuge where my mum came to seek advice and counselling whenever she became confused. She came back to the village, seeking clarity and simplicity from home whenever life seemed complicated and too much to handle. In the familiar faces of family and friends, she was made strong enough to face those difficult decisions. Cultural practices/traditions about our village do not only need to be practised but also a source of wisdom to live.

Relationships that were provided to our cultural heritage base go beyond the connections and communities. In our village, the family was not restricted to only blood relatives; it comprised neighbouring families and friends and the entire community in general. My mother took up that collective responsibility for the rest of her life. She was always the first to offer to help out, whether it be to a relative in need or to a neighbour who had trouble reaching through some bad time. She taught that it is a good Indian in the fact that one's cultural values remind them of standing by one another and being there for people in your life no matter what. That is a rich heritage instilled in her, passed down to us as one of life's most essential lessons.

With such traditions, in time, years go by, and life becomes busier, it is easy to drift away from such things and lose sight of the importance and forget whence they came. My mom never allowed that to happen. She always made us remember our heritage, lessons from the past and strength emanating from a connectedness to our own cultural identity. But above all, she would tell us that, "No matter where you inch into the world or how successful you become, your roots will guide and contribute to the wisdom."

Something which she taught me is that our roots in the culture are not only about where we come from, but they also can be a kind of resource in our future. So, every time we had to face tough decisions, she said to us, "In case of making difficult decisions at times, meditate on the value you learn from your roots."

"What has your root told you?" she used to say. "What does our culture say about this?

Leaning on that knowledge is bound to help you find an answer to your question. For her, our culture was just the compass that would help us find what we ought to do when life throws at us all those complexities, and all this with much greater clarity and purpose.

Even as modernity kept remaking the world around me, Mom's strong cultural roots stood fast like a great source of strength. For her, progress and tradition were not enemies; in fact, for her, the best and brightest in this new world could really go along with staying grounded in the old. For her, staying close to our roots has nothing to do with resistance to change. Rather, it is a process that ensures we never lose touch with ourselves while living in the light of who we were, and remain connected to such a rich cultural background, which, in a way, ruled every moment of her life choices and relationships became the norm for Daya. She had given her strength in distress, guided her in confusion, and filled her heart with joy in celebration. Her roots, she says are not merely a part of history but all of who we are; yet, they guide us as we journey through life.

With her, we learn how to stay connected with
whe   ues
that

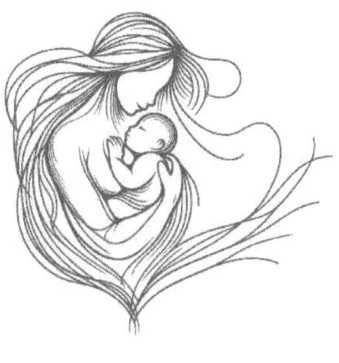

Chapter 10

Meeting Death with
Dignity- Time to Go

But that moment of enlightenment when it comes to death is one fantastic silence. It does not spring forth from a void of fear but from understanding, acceptance, and even grace. And when my mother, Daya, confronted death, facing it was really not about fighting the inevitable but embracing it. She had always been that kind of person: quiet in her strength and resilient enough to move through life's storms with remarkable resolve. Inner strength so guided her as her body failed her, both in dealing with her illness and preparations for the passing. She remained full of dignity, peace, and love for those she was soon to leave. Even as her body betrayed her, her spirit would not bend.

Do I remember the day when, with her speaking to her seven-year-old grandson Yatharth from another room, there was a follow-through of giggles and bursts of laughter? Their connection was something so special and beyond words. "I've seen Yatharth," she said to me one day, smiling. My life is now complete." Those few words spoke of deep meaning, telling how much she had valued her last moments with the little one. So strong was the connection between them that even months after she had gone, Yatharth would ask, "Can we get Grandma back for a few hours? There was something I wanted to talk to her about. His plaintive cry, "Just tell God that she is needed more here," would leave me both smiling and in tears. It was a long time in coming for him to accept that she wasn't coming back, and longer still for us all to accept her absence.

She still felt joy in her last days, be it momentary. One day, without warning, she craved for a spicy chickpea dish from the preferred restaurant she often went to. She asked my friend to bring it for her. I lost my cool when I got to know. I raised my voice and shouted at her, "You can't have that! You are not allowed to take that because of your condition! But in her usual calm, unflappable way, she smiled and said, "Just take the salt out and bring it." My friend, who knew my mother well, did not waste any time bringing her the dish. So pure, so infectious was happiness on her face that it was visible to all of us.

Even in bad health, she found joy in the smallest of things; and that is why, no matter what happens, when happiness knocks on the door, take it, because it's worth relishing. My siblings, on the other hand, just stayed with her. Helpless, they just watched her deteriorate while at the same time wanting to do more but were limited in what they could give. They could do nothing except stand by her side to give her strength whenever they possibly could and also draw it from her back to help prepare themselves for what was sure to come.

But in her body, they knew that she was giving up, yet my mother continued to emotionally support them in every quiet way as she comforted them with the same grace that had accompanied her all the way throughout life. I had actually planned to live with my elder brother and was waiting for my date schedule for a visa appointment in April 2022. I was looking forward and excited to be reunited with her in London; she was a ray of hope in this uncertain future. But that evening, it was quite different. I received a call saying that she had been admitted to the ICU on account of a sudden health breakdown. I did not waste a single minute, and I took the first available flight to Delhi, this time with the purpose that I wanted to be at her side. In my mind, I thought this was just a temporary glitch, and she'd be out of the hospital within a few days, and things would just be like before.

I carried all this optimism through the entire flight, but fate had other plans. When I was somewhere in mid-air, this lady had passed away. I did not know it was going to be like that. Just when we were landing, my wife received a call inquiring whether there could be a way they could get to me immediately. It was only after leaving the plane for Delhi that I came to know the sad news, 'Mom is no more.' As I sit back today, at least in my mind, an element of me feels that she knew somehow. She knew the man assigned the final rite was coming—and only then could she release softly.

A comfort and sorrow at once is the idea: returning from our home after her last rites was one of the most difficult things I have ever had to do. The silence filling the house was like a scream. In the silence, I could almost hear her giggling - you know, that joyful laughter which fills up all the empty halls of this house. And in my tear-covered eyes, I knew everything had changed. The house wasn't the same; neither was life.

There was an awful emptiness, a chasm no one could ever fill entirely, yet there were staccato notes of her strength and her humour, of her love, reminders she was still with us, if in spirit, to guide us through this newfound silence.

There was much inevitability to it all when she was diagnosed with liver disease in 2021. The disease had earlier snatched away two family members—to be more accurate, two members of my family: my grandmother and my mother's sister. There was no gulping denial when she got her diagnosis; instead, she seemed to have taken it as calmly as anyone could have expected, just to show me how very familiar she was with the cycles of life. I still recall her face today when we had it out to talk for the first time. And there was no panic in her eyes, just a sombre recognition of what was going to happen. Like she knew that the day was going to come and that she had simply begun to prepare herself for that journey ahead.

For the rest of us, it came as devastating news. We'd seen her face so much in her life and still come out stronger each time. She'd always have the potential to push forward. Now we knew this was different from other battles she'd been used to winning. It was something there was no chance she could possibly win. The depth of what that would mean if she did lose weighed more significantly on us but heavier on my shoulders. But the tension began to manifest in my body, and to this day, I'm baffled as to why my blood pressure came in so high-I was a plain example of my failure to cope with the reality of what was happening. Even in facing her own illness, however, she was again, in typical Daya style, more concerned about us than herself.

My mom was quite anxious about her health, but she was getting weaker by day and had me prepared much in advance asking me to begin a practice called Heartfulness, introduced by her friend. These Heartfulness meditations are meant to carry out peace and clarity for inner peace and clarity. My mother thought it was going to work for me. She wasn't planning on being cured of anything, at least not her illness, but she was very cognizant of the limited amount of time she had left. There would have to be something to dull the stress that I was under. It's almost as if she knew subconsciously that when she was gone, we would need some solace, some haven of sorts. "You must be well after I'm gone," she'd say to us as if she knew a little too well how hard it was going to be without her around. Then, almost like she was preparing me for life without her, it was almost as if she were instructing me on how to prepare myself to keep going even when she might not be around again. How selfish was her selflessness-an act of love for her children, even at death's doorstep? I am still in awe of the sheer fortitude it must have taken to love as strongly as she did in the face of death.

The last few months with her were painful and beautiful at the same time. I spent 15 days with her, which I will always treasure. Although her body was playing a trick on her, she wanted to pretend that everything was okay and continue her routine. She, of course, cooked for me three times a day, as always. She knew these were her last chances in life to take care of me the way only a mother would. Then there was something one could call heart-rupturing beautiful about moments like these, sitting at the kitchen table watching her move with slower-moving hands but still full of love and tenderness with which she fed me on more than bread alone but on memories and lessons that would serve me long after she was gone.

As the illness ran its course, she undoubtedly had little time to waste. Yet fear and despair never conceded to her; instead, she faced her mortality with an unyielding grace that has left indelible impressions on all of us. Despite her body weakening, so was not her spirit. I will never forget ten days before her death, the day she asked me if I wanted her to accompany me to the airport to see me off. Very elemental, it was in its demand, but a statement so made spoke volumes about who she was. Yet she wanted to be there for our lives, to share and seek that little moment of silence that built into each and every single minute of our bond.

It was then that we perhaps started making plans for her future; somehow, she was to spend the rest of the time with us in London. We hired a lawyer and initiated the application process for the UK settlement visa through which she would be allowed to stay with us forever. The date was finalised for April 2022 for the finalisation of her visa, and we were making all silent arrangements. But then life, as she reminds us often, has a way of making its own decisions. That is to say, it was exactly fifteen days since my mother had left this world. It was an eye-opener to cherish the memories that human planning goes just so far. We always envisioned a future where she would live with us and, therefore, we would take care of her in her final years, but fate had other plans. "We can only plan so much," she would say often. She would say, it's when it's time to go, then that's it. It was those words that I kept on having in my head now while mourning her death. She reminded us that no matter all our frantic and savage endeavors to lead our lives there are some things that just cannot be done by us.

I leave amazement at the great sagacity that my mother demonstrated in her reaction to her illness in her last months. She never once surrendered to the account of fear or malice. She accepted her fate calmly. Calmness is something that I can just aspire to; maybe my life is tough, but it's not as easy as hers. She never surrendered to life but lived for each day, connected to her friends and family, laughing over little things, letting those around her know how much they needed love and her presence. She knew that death marked life, and she never would give it the say in finality over her days.

A dying woman taught us that, even in death, there need be no fear. Death can come with dignity and perhaps peace. My mother always drew strength from our culture, and at the approaching end, she was drawing from that well of understanding. Death, in our tradition, is not the end but a transition to the eternal cycle of life. She welcomed the thought of it completely, and she prepared herself for those last days of life without fear, regret, and pain.

For those last weeks, she was not preparing herself to be gone; she was preparing us, too. She talked to every one of us not in doom-laden tones but with the same love and affection that has always defined her presence. She said she loved us, that she was proud of every one of us, and she believed most of all in the potential we might have to move on, even long after she is gone. She did not go out sad. She went out with a great sense of closure. She could bid her farewells in her quiet manner, leaving us only with memories full of joy, not of pain. Even up to now, whenever I talk to my loved ones about her last days, I am able to be full of thanksgiving and not sadness.

What my mom gave us was a gift in the way she faced her mortality. She taught us that death is not something to be abhorred; it just needs to be accepted because it is one aspect of the course of life. And for that, we learned something in the time of the end: we may let go of the option we choose, and it even comforted not only ourselves but the ones we left behind. Of course, her passing left a hollow but peaceful space as well. It was the act of giving us that window of time in which to bid our last farewells, to share in those final moments, and to witness what great strength death presents. Her legacy, though sorrowful in its sadness, was far from regretful- it was one of love, resilience, and dignity. And this is the biggest part of life: it is not measured by its length but by its depth. And in the fullness of her life, we found all the lessons we ever needed to learn. Preparing for death gave my mother the opportunity not only to give us the space in which to grieve but to equip us with tools that we'd take with us after she was gone.

She had given us memory for the strength of kindness and of indomitable belief in the importance of living life absolutely, completely, up to its last. So gracious it was to die as she had to live. And in that grace we found comfort. Yet even at the end, these words remain: "The length of a life begins when one starts to live." My mother lived-life with love, with purpose, and always close to people.

And in her final days, she showed us all that this can hold good even to dying. This is not a fight against a situation that is already over and done, but a peace in embracing it; knowing that we have lived well, loved deep, and left behind a legacy to outlive even in the long run.

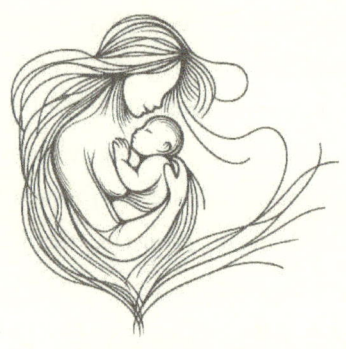

Chapter 11

The Last Conversations

There's something you never forget: the weight of the last conversations you share with somebody you love. But what do you know when you come to realise that the words, the moments you share, are finite? My last two weeks with my mother, Daya, I remember them like jammed frames, filed under an overwhelming mix of love, wisdom, and the premonition of finality. They were the epitome of her lessons in life, her reflection of the past, and a way to quietly train us on a future without her.

One evening, over dinner, she started reminiscing. "Do you know how special you were to this family when you were born? " she started. "It was after seven years of marriage that we had you. No one else in the family—your uncle brothers or your aunts—had children before you. You were the very first grandchild of my parents.

I still recall how your maternal grandmother hugged you close—that was her greatest happiness ever."

I couldn't help but joke with her, "So yes, I'm special."

Her tone turned reflective as she said, "You know how your father used to sit there and compare you with your sister Preeti. He would say he preferred your sister over you." I nodded, having been a witness to those moments that left me frustrated and restless as a child. "Something you never knew," she went on, "was that he did it on purpose." My jaw dropped in surprise. "Why?" I asked, genuinely puzzled. She said, "In our culture, boys always used to get the proper attention more than girls. When any family or friend used to come, they always took more importance of you than your sisters. Your father wanted that this inequality should never enter your thought process. He wanted you to treat your sisters as equals." It was enough for me to pause and take note of all these.

It was such a profound moment of understanding—to realise how, in the subtlest of ways, my parents had shaped values and taught lessons that I had never even been cognizant of at the time.

"I do agree with him," I said. "Preeti was and is better than me - whether it's in studies or life in general." Mother smiled softly. "That wasn't the point," she said. "Your father loved you a lot, always did." "I know, Mummy," I reassured her. "That's why I'm just like him maybe I have your courage and his goodness. That's my strength."

A few days later, she revealed another treasured memory. "Your father used to call you 'Hanuman,'" she said, referring to the legendary monkey god from Hindu mythology. "Do you know why?" I shook my head, curious. "Lord Hanuman was cursed, unaware of his own powers until someone reminded him. Your father believed that one day, when you realised your potential, you would achieve things you never imagined possible.".

Those words were her faith in me, and those were enough. Those reminded me of the amount of faith my parents had in me, even when I did not. It was as much the actions as the words that spoke for her in the last few days She returned from the market one day and asked for Rs. 200 change. "What do you want it for?" I asked. I want to buy something from her," she said. After she returned with some greens, I asked her what made her do that. She told me the story of the woman: abandoned by her son and widowed, she earned just enough to survive. Wherever you see someone needing help, help him," she said softly with action that kept it hard and firm, though gentle.

"You never know their struggles or their story," she added gently.

Helping those who are willing to fight their situation is helping yourself.

That moment proved to be one of great testimony to her untiring compassion. Even as hers was becoming worse, her heart was open to others. It was not just a lesson in kindness but in the quiet dignity of those who have had to endure hardships. Yet she had her vulnerable moments. "Sometimes I feel I have been too harsh," she said one evening, "forcing decisions on you and your sisters." I answered frankly, "Yes, you have, but we always stayed with you because we knew you did it for our own betterment. Who else would have been there for us?" My words seemed to help solace her as a proud smile appeared on her face. But as her illness progressed, so did the introspection. "You don't deserve this," she said one day, her frustration palpable. "I've made so much trouble and worry for you and your sisters. I've done what I was supposed to do here—I've seen my grandchildren. I don't need anything else." I tried to lighten the mood. "Look, you're only 60," I said, grinning.

With all the medical facilities and money we have, we will keep you alive till you are 80. After that, it's a bonus. She smiled at my optimism, and her emotions bloomed. It was a bittersweet exchange that sometimes revealed in one breath both her dread of becoming a burden and her pure love for us, even when she started losing hope, how she still managed to reassure us. "We lost Papa earlier, and now you are falling ill. I just cannot see that happening to me also," I said, my voice shaking. She looked at me with a calm strength that only she could muster. "Be with your sisters," she said. "They'll give you strength.

Unlock the powers of Hanuman within you. She left me those words as a final gift of wisdom and encouragement: "You have so much to give this world." Her last days have been tough yet a walk in grace. She stayed with her elder brother because she was waiting for her visa appointment. Suddenly, she got admitted to the ICU. I understood the message and booked a flight to Delhi at the earliest possibility, holding onto hope it was only a temporary setback. I always believed she would recover, just as she had previously. However, fate had some other plan. When I reached the middle of the journey, my mother had passed on.

The news reached my wife before me; a call from the hospital inquired if anything could reach me.

It was only when I arrived that I realised she had passed away.

I often think while thinking over that moment that she had been waiting for me. She knew it was going to be me who would perform her last rites. It is almost as if she needed that assurance before she could let go. A feeling both comforting and sorrowful. In coming home after all the final rites, the silence was just oppressive. The house felt so different now, emptier, like any emotion lives there. Yet, in this silence, I could hear her laughter, her giggles—a sound that brought comfort and tears together. Nothing will ever be that way again, but her voice, her words, and her lessons are left with us, a guiding light in the darkness. The last conversations with me reflected how she was strong, compassionate, and thoroughly bonded to her family. She left us with a legacy not just of love but of wisdom also. Through her words, she prepared the world for her absence, teaching us to draw strength from one another, help those in need, and live a purposeful life with courage. And in those last days of hers, when her body could no longer hold her upright, her spirit remained firm, reminding us that her love, her laughter, and her lessons would never completely leave us.

www.ingramcontent.com/pod-product-compliance
Ingram Content Group UK Ltd.
Pitfield, Milton Keynes, MK11 3LW, UK
UKHW040910260225
455598UK00004B/133

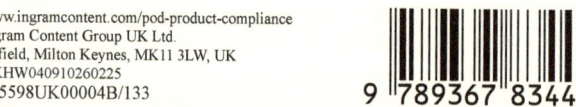